Lifted To Heaven

LIFTED To HEAVEN

A True life Experience During a Time of Death and Illness

RUTTHY WELLS

XULON PRESS

Xulon Press
2301 Lucien Way #415
Maitland, FL 32751
407.339.4217
www.xulonpress.com

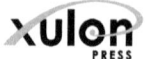

© 2018 by Rutthy Wells

All rights reserved solely by the author. The author guarantees all contents are original and do not infringe upon the legal rights of any other person or work. No part of this book may be reproduced in any form without the permission of the author. The views expressed in this book are not necessarily those of the publisher.

Unless otherwise indicated, Scripture quotations taken from the Holy Bible, New International Version (NIV). Copyright © 1973, 1978, 1984, 2011 by Biblica, Inc.™. Used by permission. All rights reserved.

Printed in the United States of America.

ISBN-13: 978-1-54564-845-2

DEDICATION

This book, Lifted To Heaven, is dedicated to:
The Father, The Son, and The Holy Spirit.
And
To My loving parents Reverend Joseph and Victoria Garcia
and to Mrs. Masako Agari, Woman of God

TABLE OF CONTENTS

Dedication................................... v
Word of Hope ix

1. A Death of Our Father...................... 1
2. Our Lives 7
3. Lifted to Heaven 9
4. Victoria's Anger........................... 13
5. Bad News of Cancer 17
6. God Heals Victoria 21

Conclusion 23
Acknowledgements........................... 25

WORD OF HOPE

*J*esus Christ promised that he would be with us in times of troubles. Our mother Victoria went through a time as a scripture says:

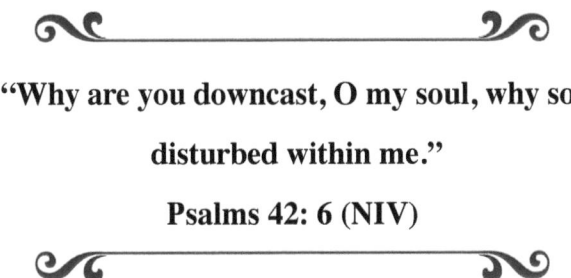

"Why are you downcast, O my soul, why so disturbed within me."

Psalms 42: 6 (NIV)

This true experience is to encourage those who are facing cancer. Victoria and I knew Lord is faithful and He will take you through a difficult time of battling cancer. Hold onto God's hand: Victoria did. Many may not understand what a person is going through with cancer, but you can to go alongside of them with kindness and tenderness. Tenderness may not be there at times; nevertheless, Jesus understands you are the help they need.

When our family was facing a time of troubles of illness and death, we reached out to relatives, our close friends, and our brethren from churched for encouragement and, most of all prayers. We sensed the kindness and love when they called us concerning our mother's illness.

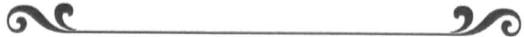

"The elders who direct the affairs of the church well are worthy of double honor, especially those whose work is preaching and teaching."
Verse 1 Timothy 5: 17 (NIV)

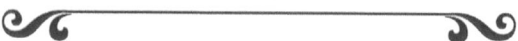

Victoria and I were thankful for Pastor Kenny Foreman and Pastor Dan Greenlee, from San Jose, California, who through their respective urban ministries had built up our faith to face this difficult time.

Chapter 1:

A Death of Our Father

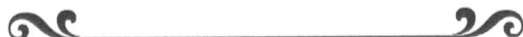

"The king was shaken. He went up to the room over the gateway and wept. As he wept, he said, "Oh my son Absalom! My son, son, my son Absalom! If only I had died instead of you-oh Absalom, my son, my son."
2 Samuel 19:33 (NIV)

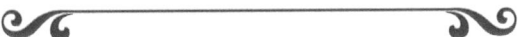

King David mourned deeply for his son Absalom. Even a king is not exempt from grief. No one can measure the depth of sorrow when a loved one dies. No one can say how long to mourn for the loss of a family member.

My mother Victoria mourned the death of our father. He died before Thanksgiving, in November of 1977. Our parents had been married for fifty-three years. Together they had pastored four

Hispanic Methodist Churches. They were like brother and sister in a close relationship.

A telephone call came while I worked in Pasadena. My mother told me that my father was seriously ill and I should come home to Stockton to help her. My position as a secretary was becoming too complicated with work details; I decided to give my notice to quit. My father was needing my help.

When I arrived in Stockton where my parents lived, I rushed into my parents bedroom. Our dad was in bed. He looked at me; his face was so pale, almost white, his lips were chapped badly. His forehead was hot with a fever as I touched it. I said, "Dad, can you get up? We have to get you to a doctor."

He answered weakly, "I can..." and as he stood up, he almost collapsed in my arms. I assisted him step by step into the living room. Quickly I made a decision to take him to the doctor's office. My mother called Dr. Sidney Mallet right away and told him my dad was being rushed to his office. Our neighbor, Mr. Brown, a strong man, helped me put him in my car. I told my mother to rest and sleep. She was very exhausted. For two months she had been hired as a floor lady at a local cannery.

At the doctor's office, the doctor was waiting for him with a gurney, and was rushed into the office. I left him there, and returned home to help my mother. I needed to rest and to pray. As I prayed, I realized that I was telling God to heal our dad. Crazy thoughts were going through my mind. We as a family had never had a serious illness, especially one that looked serious enough for death. Our dad as a pastor had officiated at many funerals of our relatives and now it might be our turn to experience a death. I called my brothers and sisters to let them know dad was sick and was in Saint Joseph's Hospital in Stockton.

After one hour I was informed that my dad had been transferred immediately to the hospital. After my mother and I rested, we went to the hospital. The doctor gave us the diagnosis. The lupus disease had spread all over his organs and there was no cure for him. We learned that lupus was an autoimmune disorder. Our dad had an advanced case of the disease. The nursing staff would make him as comfortable as they could. The bad news was that my dad had a short time to live.

At the hospital, visitors, friends, relatives, all lined up to visit him. When some friends told him that God would heal him, he would answer calmly, "Pray for yourselves. The Lord has told me I am going home."

My sister Ann and my brother Joe, came to help my mother. I was ill with the flu and because dad was infectious, I could not see him. My brother and sister came at the right time to take care of our mother. I knew God was with our dad and was being treated like a king.

After I was feeling better from the flu, my sisters and my brother went to see dad. We had to wear hospital protective gowns, gloves, and a mask over our mouths. Dad was contagious after surgery. The doctors informed us that dad had been bleeding from his lungs and surgery was necessary to stop the bleeding. When we entered the room we began singing uplifting songs. All of us had been Born-Again and filled with the Spirit in 1976. Before he died he told my sister Esther that he kept hearing a hymn in his spirit; it just kept going on nonstop.

At midnight we had gathered at home and we were praising God. We worshipped God who had given us a good husband and a good father. My sister Esther remained at the hospital. My heart told me to help them all worship God; even in the midst the tears and sorrow. Then I remembered to call Mr. Irvin Thomas in Selma, California who had known my father for the many funerals he had officiated in his mortuary. Mr. Thomas had promised our family that he would pick up our dad's body from the hospital when he died. Mr. Thomas came early in the morning hours and picked up our dad's body. We will never forget the kindness of this man.

All of us were mourning the death of our General. Our dad had been the strength of our family. He always was telling us that he would protect us from anyone that would hurt us in any way. Our dad was six foot eleven inches tall and muscled; could do head-stands easily.

Overwhelmed with his death, I took time and entered the garage to be alone. I cried and asked God a lot of questions. After a few minutes the Holy Spirit said to me, "Are you through crying?" Then even before I answered, the Lord told me that my dad had been ready for heaven when we were younger. But because we were still young, God had mercy on us and did not take dad then to heaven. The Lord continued to say to me, "Now get up, wipe your tears, and know that the same God your dad served, now it is you and your siblings to continue the work of the Lord."

We held his funeral in Selma, California, where he first began his ministry as a young pastor. Many relatives and friends from Selma, Stockton, and San Jose attended the celebration of life for our dad. Returning to Stockton, we mourned together as a family. A few days later we would be celebrating Thanksgiving. Thanksgiving was not at this time important to us—our dad was missing. Gabriel our dad's nine year old grandson was having a difficult time with his grandfather's death. At the onset, of his grandpas illness, he would sit and watch his friend and take deep sighs. One morning he burst into the kitchen as we were having breakfast. He was excited about his dream. He said, "I know where grandpa is… I saw him dressed in a white gown hugging Jesus." From that time on, happiness seemed to be reflect in everything he said. My mother was grieving and very exhausted. Yet none of us were really seeing how tired and worn out she was because we were all mourning our father.

Chapter 2:
Our Lives

When I got over the flu, I returned to the Bay Area, San Jose, and shared my sister's apartment. Before my dad's death, I had applied at an employment agency for another job. God knew I needed another job. I interviewed and the engineering bosses liked my secretarial skills and I was hired. The church were I had been a member before I moved to Los Angeles became my church again.

On the weekends I would pack some clothes and went to Stockton to console my mother. My siblings did not go every weekend as I did. Then I stopped going every weekend because the dense fog was too dangerous for me drive to Stockton. In February of 1978, my mother was not doing well. She sounded depressed and still mourning. She would call me at work and her tone was one of loneliness. I remembered how she had always been surrounded by brethren of the church and church activities. Now there was no one and to top it all, her two best friends died too. My burden for her grew quickly. I decided to pack some clothes and at the end of

Friday's work day, I drove to Stockton. I would read the bible, sing hymns, and cook meals for her. I did whatever I could do to keep her spirit alive. I felt she would die if I didn't come to her aid. On Sunday nights I would go home to San Jose.

One Sunday night I was late coming back to San Jose. All was fine until I came to the Altamont Pass. This Pass was familiar to me. No problem. However, as I continued to drive I encountered a thick pocket of fog. In the fog I tried to follow the rear lights of the car ahead of me. In a second I lost that car and did not know if I was in the middle lane or the far right lane. I was frightened and kept saying, "Jesus, Jesus, Jesus, I need your help!" Anything could have happened to me. Exhaustion, fog giving me a sensing of drifting, I needed Jesus's help.

Jesus heard my cry because in a few seconds the fog lifted. I sighed with relief. With my left hand I brushed my tears away. The drive from Stockton took close to two hours. I arrived at my apartment close to midnight. Parked my car; took the elevator to the third floor; entered my room. My sister Ann shared the apartment with me. She was fast asleep and I tried to not make noise to wake her up. Quickly I threw my clothes on a chair and put on a nightgown. I was overcome with exhaustion and literally dropped on my bed like a log. In a few minutes I went into a deep sleep.

Chapter 3:

LIFTED TO HEAVEN

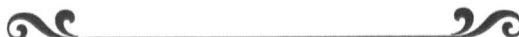

"I know a man in Christ who fourteen years
ago was caught up in the third heaven.
Whether it was in the body or out of the body
I do not know–God knows. And I know that
this man whether in the body or apart from the
body I do not know–God knows–was caught
up in Paradise."

2 Corinthians 12:1-4 (NIV)

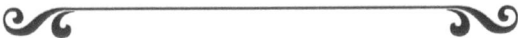

In my sleep, I began to experience queasiness in my stomach. Then I felt lightness come over me that made me feel like I was floating. I was unable to stop the feeling. The floating took me above my bed and as I was in the air, I saw myself lying on my bed. I glanced upward and I went right through the ceiling.

I had no control on what was happening to me.

Then I went through what seemed like a dark tunnel for a few seconds. At the end of the tunnel I saw a bright light. Then two angels were carrying me in a stretcher with a brilliant white fluffy thin fitted covering below me. Each angel was at each end of the stretcher.

As they carried me, I glanced at a bright gold, tall building and the tops of more buildings though not as tall. Yet they glowed as well. To me, it was a city that did not have a sun. The angels kept carrying me somewhere. I was not afraid all this time.

Then we entered a lovely park with trees, bushes, along the path. I saw people, their backs to me, praying on their knees; inside shelters. They did not turn around to see me.

Then at some point the angels laid me down. It seemed like a second when Jesus appeared. I knew who he was and heard his voice. He called the disciples saying, "Quickly, my sister has to return home." Jesus positioned them around me. I remember Moses was there holding my head. Saint Paul was at my right holding my hand. They began to pray powerfully for me. Then Jesus laid his head on my bosom and stayed there for a few seconds. I felt the warmth of a loving Jesus.

The angels lifted me up and carried me again. They laid me down again and it seemed like I was standing and looking at the universe. I heard the voice of the Lord like the sound of many waters. The amplification of His voice was astonishing from one end to the other end of the universe.

I woke up at 4:30 a.m. when I felt my spirit just drop into my body. I was in my bed and I began to cry.

The next day I was able to go to work and had incredible energy. I felt like I was walking on air. One friend, a spiritual co-worker, Leonard Van Arsdale looked at me and said, "Ruth what happened to you? You look like you've had a spiritual vision!" He said he could see it on my face. So I told him what happened to me. He praised God and hugged me.

Many co-workers heard my experience and were inspired. As I was hired to work at another company, some co-workers asked me to relate to them my spiritual experience. I always gave God the Glory.

Chapter 4:
VICTORIA'S ANGER

A year later, all of us continued with our lives. My siblings and I remained in San Jose in our homes and in our jobs. My mother remained in Stockton, living by herself. Sometimes she had young women that shared her home for a few weeks or months. Often they helped our mom with monetary help, or just being there for her. It wasn't easy for her to adjust to living by herself without our father.

My job in San Jose was good until the company went through a reorganization. I left the company in good standing and sought temporary jobs with various employment agencies. I always had a job, because I had good skills as a secretary.

At times my mother would call me at work. She sounded very monotone and I knew she had lost more weight by eating skimpy meals. Some of her words caused me concern. She said, "Those people in bars sound like they're having a good time; I should join them." Another time she said, "I wish I could be like them–lively and all." I was concerned about her loneliness and somber words.

How could I help my mother who I loved dearly. I prayed and thanked God for He answered my prayer.

My mother had sought out a former retired Pastor who had known my father. They had met at an Annual Methodist Conference. When she met with him, she confessed to him that she had anger towards God. Her anger was for taking her husband and some close church friends. After talking to Pastor Combes she later told me that he was, "Very kind and gentle." He also told her that anger was a Godgiven emotion. "Victoria," he said, "you can have anger, but you can't stay angry." She came home and recounted that the visit had helped her, but she still was angry at God.

One night, the Lord gave me a dream:

> *My mother had gone to a chapel, in a cemetery, to visit dad's grave. Dusk was setting in and she had not come out of the chapel. The Lord was telling me that my mother needed to leave the chapel, for the gate would close soon. I rode a bicycle as fast as I could. I needed to get her out of that chapel. I reached her in time and we rode out, double back, just as the gate closed behind us.*

With the help of the Holy Spirit, I interpreted the dream. The Lord was telling me that my mother was dying ahead of her time. My life again was on hold as I visited her during this time.

Chapter 5:

BAD NEWS OF CANCER

Victoria had gone to an appointment with her doctor. There she discovered that she had lymphoma cancer. She called each one of us and was very upset.

I was working at General Electric and had a good secretarial position. Confusion and bosses that were not getting along helped me to make a decision to terminate my job and move back to Stockton. I moved in with my mother and helped her with her bout of cancer. My trust in God strengthened me to know He would help both of us deal with the cancer.

My mom was referred to Dr. Dighe Pradsad, MD. He was a well known physician, and was to be in charge of treating her cancer. He let us know how the treatment would be and addressed the dangers of it as well.

Victoria doubted the doctor's counsel on taking chemotherapy intravenously for several months. She was still angry at God for letting her husband die. And adding chemotherapy treatments to was not agreeable to her. Yet there was a glimmer of hope in the treatment.

First, she had to undergo surgery on her tonsil on the left side of her throat. The cancer was on that tonsil. Our family worked together to get her to eat healthy meals to keep her strong for the surgery. Her faith was still strong. She kept asking for all her grandchildren. Some were living in Montana, Nancy, her granddaughter was living in Japan with her husband. Nancy was very concerned about her grandmother Victoria.

Victoria underwent the surgery. All went well and she recovered quickly. The doctor waited a few weeks to start the chemotherapy treatments. After resting for two weeks after surgery, she was angry to start the treatments. Her anger was very evident to all the family and friends who were close to her. Many were praying for her and gave her words of encouragement.

All of my brothers, sisters, and I were working in the Bay Area. We took turns checking in on her after the surgery. The first chemo treatments went well. About the fourth treatment, her vein collapsed and she would have to get the treatment another way. Dr. Dighe made a decision to make an incision right in the middle of her chest. He inserted a tube so that he could keep the treatment going.

Our prayers brought in a friend Eva, who knew our mom from the church that our father had pastored. God was timely in bringing her to assist our mother. She had a nursing background. Eva was a blessing as she gave our mother encouragement, and she made good meals for her. Eva also prayed and provided spiritual support. These times were full of disappointment for our mom. She began to lose her hair. She would look in the mirror; mumbling followed with words of anger and criticism about her condition. I learned to be patient with her and tried not to overreact to her anger.

What could I say, I was incapable of understanding what she was going through in her illness. Now she was almost bald and ashamed to go out to do errands. Eva was there to drive her to more doctor appointments. At my suggestion we brought her a head scarf that looked like a cap with white straps to tie behind the cap or around her neck. We chose a colorful one.

One day she decided to mow the lawn with and old lawn mower that we had in the garage. This was a day when she needed someone to be around. As she mowed the lawn, the blades struck a small stone and it bounced and hit her right in the chest where the tube was inserted. She was bleeding; Eva quickly to get her to the ER. My younger sister Sally and her young sons, Gabriel and Jerome, were living with her when this accident occurred. They were helping and trying to keep her calm.

Cancer had spread to her head and a big lump surfaced. Her condition was Lymphoma. She counted the lumps on her left arm that she could feel with her hand. Eva told her there were seven lumps. The largest was on the top of her head. Dr. Dighe told her she would have to get radiation treatments after the final chemo treatment. This time she told him she would wait because her home was being remodeled. The city of Stockton moved her into a small home while her home was being remodeled.

My concern was to help keep my mom's faith strong. I kept praying and reading the word of God to her. I made good meals and even motivated her to eat when she had no taste for food because of the radiation.

We were dealing with several lumps on her left arm and the big lump on the top of her head. Her hair was growing back and it looked even healthier than before.

I looked into the books of Christians who wrote about spiritual healing. I was not one who knew about healing, I wanted to learn all that I could. We had been a Pastor's family, did the work of the Lord, but we never knew about the Holy Spirit and the ministry of healing. In San Jose, I attended Faith Tabernacle Church with Pastor Kenny Foreman. I served as a Sunday school teacher. Pastor Kenny Foreman had been a good preacher on signs, wonders, and miracles. He as a young boy had been healed from a grave sickness. I remembered a powerful message he gave on what to do in "The Eye of a Storm." A book written by Kenneth Hagin told me clearly that my mother could be healed. I read it to her and together our faith grew stronger.

Chapter 6:
GOD HEALS VICTORIA

That night, she was worn out and tired. I looked at her and said, "Mom, you need to tell God what you want to do. If you want to go to Heaven, it's fine with us your family, but if you stay, you need to tell us how to help you." She did not answer me and instead went into her bedroom and closed the door.

Around 3:30 a.m., my mom woke up and started shouting, "I was perspiring a lot and my bumps, they're gone!" I got up from my bed and walked to her room. The big lump on her head was completely gone. The other lumps on her left arm were gone as well. My mom was excited and amazed at her healing. She had gone into her bedroom and had been on her knees praying to God and whatever she said, God touched her and healed her.

Even though she knew she was healed, she went back for another radiation treatment. I knew she did not need that treatment anymore for she had received a miracle from Jesus.

My mom and I went to a spiritfilled Assembly of God Church in downtown Stockton. After a few visits Pastor Eugene Laurence baptized her. She was filled with the Holy Ghost, spoke in the heavenly language.

For three years she went around Stockton telling her friends and people of her miracle and testifying that Jesus had healed her.

At that time, we still lived in the home where she had received the miracle. I was lifted to Heaven by Jesus.

The Lifted to Heaven Again:

Queasiness came over me as I was sleeping. I then felt as my body was being lifted. I was Jesus; he took my hand and held it tightly. We were walking in the air above homes. It was dark. I stayed very close to Jesus. Somewhere I could hear the shrill voices of demonic activity, but I held tight to His hand. I saw people sleeping in their homes. There were no roofs. We kept going above homes and I saw more sleeping people.

We stopped above a rich looking home with a nice patio and swimming pool, but no one was there. Then as I turned, I was back in my bed.

There were no words between Jesus and I as we walked. Later I knew that these were the people I would be ministering to in my life. And it is and has been as Jesus showed me.

Conclusion

*Y*et, every day I give thanks to Jesus and God for extending my life. My mother's healing was a blessed time for all of us. Since then I have ministered to many in hospitals, convalescent hospitals, and prayed in my church as an altar worker. I have seen many miracles since that experience and I give thanks and Glory to God.

Then too, many of our pastors who gave us powerful messages during difficult times we would remember. So our family was encouraged by Pastor Kenny Foreman, Pastor Dan Greenlee, Evangelist Dwight Thompson, who went through a time of sorrow when his younger brother died. All these sermons and their words had built our family up spiritually to endure a time of our Storm.

Our mother Victoria died on February 15, 2006. God granted her twenty more years. Her death was reported as an undiagnosed illness. To our amazement, she was not speaking in English several days before her death. She spoke in what was a Heavenly language that was accompanied with her smile.

LIFTED TO HEAVEN

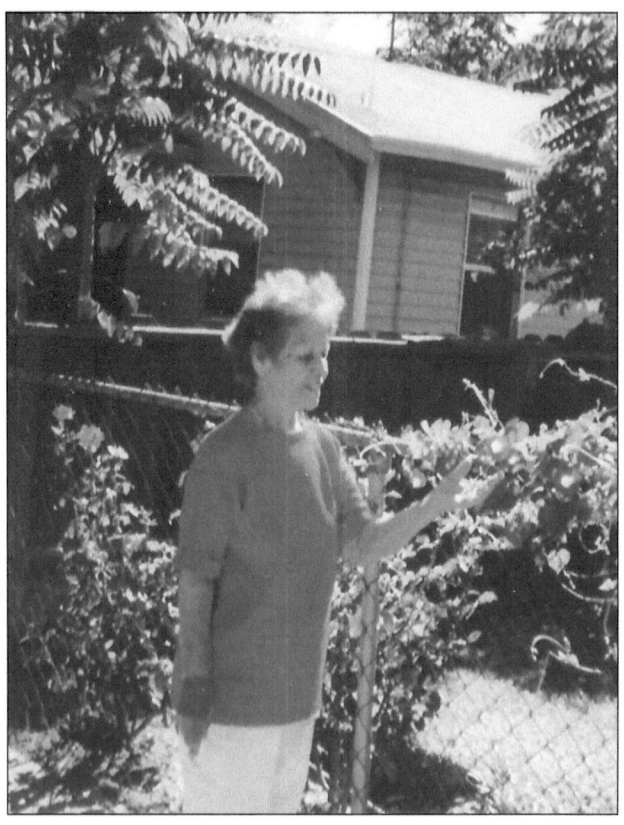

Victoria is enjoying her morning glories after being healed.

ACKNOWLEDGEMENTS

The Gracia family thank all friends who supported us in our time of sorrow and death.

Mrs. Masako Agari, a faithful woman of God who interceded for our family. She is Ninety-eight years of age and lives in Stockton, California.

Pastor Curtis Holland, Foursquare Church, Stockton CA. He uplifted prayers and church members kept in touch with Victoria at his request.

Mrs. Guillermina Manzo and her family, Sal and Mona Acosta, and Daisy. Lupe Trejo (deceased) all loving neighbors from Stockton CA.

Don and Katherine Altnow, Lodi CA, who gave Victoria their love and support.

Leslie Ann Altnow, Lodi CA, was a special young lady that brought joy to our mother.

Victoria's grandchildren: Nancy, Jackie, Albert Jr., Gabriel, Jerome, Joe III, Jeff, Joshua, Diana, Jesse, Michelle, all were special grandchildren, loved by Victoria.

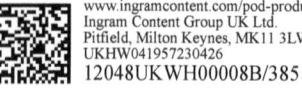